The Intermittent Fasting Weight Loss Formula

How To Lose Weight Fast, Keep it Off & Renew
The Mind, Body & Spirit Through Fasting,
Smart Eating & Practical Spirituality - Volume 2

ROBERT DAVE JOHNSTON

Published by:

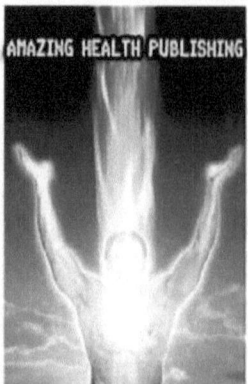

If you are interested in reading the next volume, follow Rob on Twitter @RobDaveJohnston

Copyright

Disclaimer & Legal Notices

The health-related information and suggestions contained in any of the books or written material mentioned above are based on the research, experience and opinions of the Author and other contributors. Nothing herein should be misinterpreted as actual medical advice, such as one would obtain from a Physician, or as advice for self-diagnosis or as any manner of prescription for self-treatment.

Neither is any information herein to be considered a particular or general cure for any ailment, disease or other health issue. The material contained within is offered strictly and solely for the purpose of providing Holistic health education to the general public. Persons with any health condition should consult a medical professional before entering this or any fasting, weight loss, detoxification or health related program.

Even if you suffer from no known illness, we recommend that you seek medical advice before starting any fasting, weight loss and/or detoxification program, and before choosing to follow any advice given this book. For any products or services mentioned or suggested in this book, you should read all packaging and instructions, as no substance, natural or drug, can be guaranteed to work in everyone.

Information and statements regarding dietary supplements, products or services mentioned in this book many not have been evaluated by the Food and Drug Administration and are not intended to diagnose, treat, cure, or prevent any disease. Never disregard or delay in seeking professional medical advice because of something you have read in this book.

Nothing that you read in this book should be regarded as medical or health advice. If you do anything recommended in this book, without the supervision of a licensed medical doctor, you do so at your own risk. Not recommended for persons with any health related condition unless supervised by a qualified health practitioner.

Because there is always some risk involved in any health-related program, the Author, Publisher and contributors assume no responsibility for any adverse effects or consequences resulting from the use of any suggested preparations or procedures described in any of the books or other written materials associated with the website FitnessThroughFasting.com. The author reserves the right to alter and update his opinions based on new conditions at any time.

Dedication

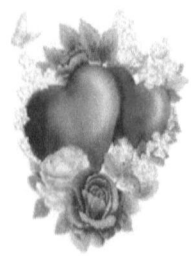

This series of books are dedicated to my mother Sonia Noemi, without whom I would not even be alive today. I love you mom. Thank you for never losing faith in me and supporting me, even when everything seemed hopeless and everyone else had given up on me. I owe you everything. I could collect all of the precious stones on this earth and lay them on your lap, and even still, I would not even come close to giving back to you all that you have given me.

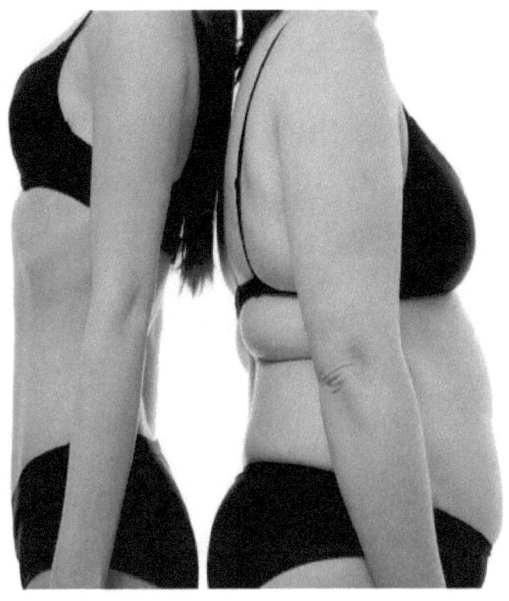

"No matter how busy your daily schedule may be, intermittent fasting gives you plenty of options to lose weight fast, detoxify and give your health a massive, positive boost."

Chapter 1
Stop & Go Weight Loss

Welcome to the world of intermittent fasting (**IF**). In this book I want to give you a comprehensive look at what intermittent fasting is, how you can lose 15 pounds (or more) every month as well as detoxify, and what you can expect to go through while you're fasting.

In Volume 3 of this series, **How to Lose 30 Pounds (or more) in 30 Days With Juice Fasting**, I provided a very aggressive weight loss and cleansing plan. Here, I give you another option that, while it may not produce weight loss as fast as with juice fasting, **still gives you a huge push forward toward your goals**.

For some people, losing weight consistently is more important than the speed. Or perhaps you are very busy and simply don't have time to be preparing juices. Whatever your situation may be, intermittent fasting will help you to lose a great deal of weight very fast (faster than with any traditional diet), while also giving your digestive system the time to detox and heal. It is a very powerful method that can literally transform your life. I know this because it totally has changed my entire view of food, eating, weight loss and health. I will give you tons of options so that, no matter what your schedule may be, you can benefit from the amazing benefits that (**IF**) always provides.

What matters most is that you have the **willingness to give this a shot to the very best of your ability**. You don't have to follow my instructions to perfection or set any fasting records. But I do want you to realize that intermittent fasting is not an '*overnight*' or '*miracle*' cure. It will require you to **roll up your sleeves and do some work**. If you are persistent and realistic, I have no doubt that you will accomplish great things.

It is also important for me to emphasize that fasting by itself will not suffice. Even though (**IF**) produces very fast weight loss, it is important that you realize the need for permanent eating habit changes. You can fast for months and lose lots of weight. However, if you return to poor eating habits, then I guarantee you that the weight loss will be short-lived. I am not interested in writing *'another weight loss book'* that, in the end, solves nothing. I want to give you *'the meat'* that you will need to get the weight off, and **<u>KEEP IT OFF</u>**.

To that end, in addition to the **(IF)** strategies, I will also give you a basic dietary foundation to follow once the fast is over.

For a detailed diet and instructions, I strongly recommend that you read <u>Volume 1</u> of the series **The Permanent Weight Loss Diet.**' That book gives you the specific diet that I have been following for years, and which has allowed me to lose more than 100 pounds and keep them off.

Intermittent Fasting: Definition

Dictionary.com says: in·ter·mit·tent [in-ter-mit-nt] (adjective) means:

• Stopping or ceasing for a time; alternately ceasing and beginning again: Example: an intermittent pain.
• Alternately functioning and not functioning or alternately functioning properly and improperly.
• (of streams, lakes, or springs) recurrent; showing water only part of the time.

These definitions have one thing in common: they refer to an act that is **PARTIAL** and happens only **SOME OF THE TIME**. That is precisely what **(IF)** is all about. You fast for a little bit of time; you return to eating for a little bit of time. It is a *'stop and go'* structure of weight loss.

This **ON** and **OFF** process can be repeated daily, weekly and/or monthly. Better yet, it is **NO LESS** effective than an extended uninterrupted fast, **AS LONG** as you keep a clean diet when you eat. To be sure, the weight loss won't be as quick and dramatic as it would be during a total juice or water fast. But you **WILL** lose weight, and it will be much faster than with a traditional diet. **(IF)** is also an excellent way to cleanse the digestive system over a period of months. So if you have been looking for an effective (*and proven*) way to lose weight fast and improve your health, then **(IF)** can definitely help you to get there.

Time Is On Your Side

Intermittent fasting is just like that oldie but goodie song by the Rolling Stones where Mick Jagger sings - "Tiiiiime is on my side." **(IF)** gives you the flexibility to "*sneak in*" times of fasting anytime during a day, week or month. **(IF)** can be as simple as skipping one meal daily.

The bottom line is this: With **(IF)**, time is on your side! If you have a lot of weight to lose and/or have eaten poorly for years, it is easier *(at first)* to complete a partial fast than it is to do an extended non-interrupted one. Little baby steps eventually add up to a mile. Those are some of the reasons why this "alternating" method of fasting is becoming increasingly popular. I get tons of emails from people inquiring about **(IF)**. In this book I hope to answer most, if not all of the questions you may have.

In short, (IF) removes all excuses that people have for <u>NOT</u> taking action and losing excess weight. Whether you have time or not, are busy or not or whatever... (IF) can help you to shed the blubber fast. No matter what your schedule or goals may be, (IF) can be customized.

Chapter 2
Calorie Restriction Benefits

In recent times, more information has come to light about (**IF**), which can also be referred to as <u>calorie restriction</u> (**CR**). <u>Eating less</u> has been found to extend lifespan and increase resistance to age-related diseases in lab rats and monkeys.

Research indicates that calorie restriction via (**IF**) enhances the cardiovascular system by decreasing risk factors for coronary artery disease. Calorie restriction through (**IF**) also supports brain functions by **decreasing risk factors for stroke such as high blood pressure**. The beneficial effects of (*CR*) are directly linked to the reduction of what is known as <u>oxidative stress</u>.

To put it simply, oxidative stress means that the body has become inundated with <u>free radicals and toxins</u> picked up through food, air and water. Oxidative stress fosters a build-up of toxins because the body is unable to process them quickly enough. And regular (**IF**) can minimize and even vanquish this harmful phenomena.

Furthermore, studies on calorie restriction indicate that (**IF**) has the same effects on the brain and cardiovascular system as those received from physical exercise! To put it simply, this means that the detoxification, weight loss and overall purification attained through intermittent fasting are similar to the ones attained via regular, vigorous exercise. Imagine that!

It took me 25 years to come out of my prison of obesity and toxicity. Unfortunately, I didn't have support or anybody to help and give me directions. If I had, I am certain I wouldn't have had to endure so many years of misery. Nevertheless, I take comfort in the fact that my bitter experience can now be used to help others.

Here's the bottom line: One year of your life dedicated to (**IF**) (*regardless of the length of each fast*) can have a dramatic impact and **shake the foundations of your entire existence**. I know of people who have gone from overweight and hopeless to vibrant, dynamic and inspirational personalities that make a positive impact in the life of others. They did this through a solid structure of (**IF**).

Some have changed careers, moved to a different country, become public speakers, spiritual leaders, public servants, world travelers, authors etc... anybody can increase the list. Others have literally been healed of illness, lost hundreds of pounds and avoided premature death. I give you this introductory information so that you can internalize the magnitude of what you are now undertaking. While fast weight loss is one of the most sought-after benefits of this practice, now you can see that (**IF**) has a world of benefits that will touch every aspect of your life.

Chapter 3
How to Use This Book

Let's take a look at the *'plan of action'* that we'll be following in this book. First and foremost I will talk about the <u>different types of fasting</u> methods that you can practice. I will give you a general idea of how much weight one can expect to lose with each one. We'll take a look at <u>what the body goes through when we fast</u>, how the process works and the *'detox'* symptoms that you may experience. As part of your pre-fasting preparation, I will give you a list of banned foods for you to start eliminating right away. I definitely want to start challenging you to make changes quickly so that you can see results as quickly as possible.

Getting Results

I gather that you purchased this book because **you want to produce tangible results**. So I am not going to pull any punches. I am going to give you a step-by-step plan and <u>push you to take action</u>. There may be some moments when I will be blunt and you *'may not like me.'* You'll get over it.

I can tell you right from the start: Achieving long-term success with (IF) will require you to **let go of the trash that you may have been eating all this time**. If you are planning to fast and do nothing else, then that won't cut it. **Fasting only to return to eating junk is a waste of time**. You might as well throw this book away for give it to someone who is willing to go all the way.

I am not saying that you have to be *'perfect.'* We all stumble and fall short of our goals sometimes. What I <u>AM</u> asking you is to enter into this with a **sincere desire and willingness to improve your relationship with food**. Don't worry, I will give you some dietary tips that will help get you started. All that I ask is that you remain <u>open-minded and willing to take action</u>.

Do that, and you will certainly experience notable weight loss and improvements in your health. And nothing makes my day more than knowing that you reached your goals. That is the sole purpose of every book that I write. Helping you to go the distance and live a life of **optimum health and personal freedom**.

Once we look at the *'banned foods,'* I will present you with the **FIVE (IF) METHODS FOR ULTIMATE WEIGHT LOSS AND HEALTH.** We will look at each of them individually and I will explain to you how they work.

You will have a chance to peruse the information and select which one fits best with your lifestyle and current schedule. Then I will walk you through a sample daily schedule of intermittent fasting. In it, I will give you tips, ideas and suggestions on what to do daily while you are fasting to get through hunger and detox symptoms.

Furthermore, I will provide detailed instructions on how to break the fast appropriately and returning to a clean diet. All in all, this book will give you the A-Z of intermittent fasting. I will throw in the kitchen's sink to make sure that you get everything that you need to get the job done.

Fasting Journal

If you have read any of my other books, then you know that I always insist on the importance of keeping a fasting journal during this process. This is important because I will be asking you to take notes and write your thoughts and feelings as we move along.

Please do not just grab any piece of crap notebook that you may have laying around. Go out and actually purchase a nice-looking journal that you can use as your 'special place' in which to write about your journey with fasting.

I have journals going back five, 10 ... 12 years. I cherish them all as they contain information about me... where I was, what I was thinking etc. That information is invaluable to me because it allows me to see where I have made progress, where I may still be stuck... and what are the key vulnerabilities in my life and personality that I have to stay on top of.

So please: purchase this journal. You won't regret it. From now on I am going to assume that you have it. If you are serious about going all the way with (IF), then I urge you to follow my instructions. I have been down this road many times before and know what works and what doesn't. Stick with me. You are not alone!

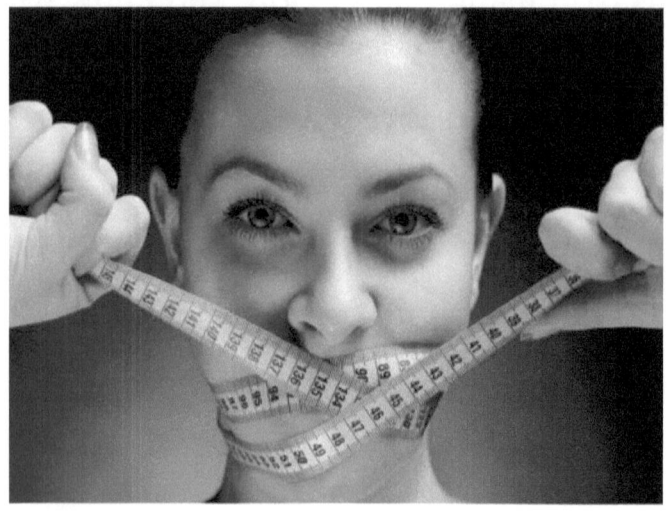

"Practice is the key to fasting. The more you practice fasting... the longer and longer periods you go without eating, the stronger your <u>mental muscles</u> will become to resist hunger and detox symptoms."

Chapter 4
Types of Fasting

The first step I want to take is to go through the different 'methods' of fasting. It is very important that you become thoroughly acquainted with them so that you can decide which one you want to practice. You may have already picked up with this book knowing what type of fast you are going to do. Nonetheless, I ask you to indulge so that we can be on the same page.

Juice Fasting. is the most popular kind of fasting. With juice fasting, you extract the juice from fruits and veggies using an appliance known as a juicer. During whatever period of time you are fasting, you drink only the juice and water. No solid food is ingested.

Here's my personal juice fasting recipe: tomatoes, broccoli, watercress, apples, pears, strawberries and blueberries - the liquid mixed in a gallon-jug and topped with water. I use this mixture regularly to do three and seven-day spurts of juice fasting. Juice fasting is the easiest kind of fasting.

I say *'easy'* guardedly because, in truth, no type of fasting is easy. What I mean is that, since the body will be receiving nourishment from the fruits and veggies, juice fasting is not as harsh as fasting with only water (*which I will talk about below*). Juice fasting is extremely powerful because the body receives a massive jolt of amazing nutrients.

Overall, weight loss with juice fasting in the first 10 days can fluctuate from 7 to 20 pounds (*depending on health and body makeup*), and then settles on **one-to-two pounds per day**. Many people with chronic illnesses have used juice fasting for healing and to support traditional (and harsher) treatments. I myself relied on juice fasting for several years when I was fighting a liver condition that hit me as a result of years of poor eating and destructive living.

Water Fasting is basically exactly that: drinking water only - not eating anything. Typically, weight loss while water fasting ranges from 1 to 20 pounds (*or more*) in the first seven days. I am talking here of a straight water fast. In other words, not eating for seven days straight. I will give you (IF) weight loss figures later once we enter into that discussion. After the first seven days of straight water fasting, you can usually expect to lose anywhere from one-to-two pounds daily.

Some people lose as many as three and four pounds daily with water fasting. But that isn't the norm. **One-to-two pounds per day is the average that I see in 95% of the cases**. It is important to note that as much as 30% of the weight lost in the first seven days of water fasting is comprised of water weight. Once the body has finished detoxifying (*about 9 to 11 days*), the weight lost becomes 98% fat and around 2% muscle tissue. Specific weight loss figures depend depends on body makeup and overall health.

Absolute Fasting. (*also known as dry fasting*) is the **grand daddy of all fasting methods**. It is about going through a period of time without drinking water **OR** eating. There are two types of absolute fasting: *soft and hard*. Soft dry fasting is where you do not drink water or eat anything but **DO** take showers or go swimming. In other words, you can have contact with water *'on the outside'* only. Yes, you could *'sing in the rain'* if you wanted. :-)

The other form of absolute fasting is the 'hard' type. Hard dry fasting is where you do not drink any water or eat, **OR** have any kind of external contact with water (*shower, swimming, singing in the rain etc..*) Dry fasting, by far, is the fasting type that produces the most weight loss in the least amount of time. The average is 20 pounds in three days. However, as is the case with water fasting, most of the weight that you lose will be water weight. In this case, water weight will likely amount to 70% of the weight lost because the body actually goes into dehydration.

There are some who maintain that absolute fasting could cure the common cold if practiced when symptoms first emerge. I have read cases of people who have done an absolute fast for three-to-five days and were reportedly cured of life-long allergic reactions and conditions. The process behind the healing power of dry fasting is that, since the body is not receiving food or hydration, overall bodily functions slow down to a minimum. Consequently, it is believed, the immune system has a much greater amount of resources to seek and destroy all sort of sickness - even viruses.

While with juice and water fasting bodily functions slow down considerably, **a dry fast reduces them much further**. This deeper reduction in body functions, it is believed, gives the immune system ultra healing capacity. Sort of like being stuck in a traffic jam for hours and then, suddenly, having all of the traffic disappear and having the road all to yourself. Since you no longer have to share the road with any other vehicles, you are free to speed up and go as fast as you want.

I completed a 72-hour 'soft' dry fast some years ago and can tell you that it is probably among the hardest things I've ever done. You can read more about my dry fasting experience at the main website **FitnessThroughFasting.com**. Dry fasting is dangerous and should not be practiced unless one is **VERY** experienced in fasting and calorie restriction.

Which Type of Fast Should I Do?

If you are experienced with fasting, then probably you already have a plan of action. However, I recommend that you stick to juice fasting if you are new. In that time, you will learn a lot about how your body reacts when calories are restricted. You may experience mild to medium detox symptoms. You may experience harsh symptoms, like I did.

Practice is the key to fasting. The more you practice fasting... the longer and longer periods you go without eating, the stronger your <u>mental muscles</u> will become to resist hunger and detox symptoms. Initially, stick to what is easiest. You can work your way up from there. This is not a race and there is nobody around *'measuring'* how weak or strong you are. **Be persistent but also be patient with yourself,** especially if you have never used a juicer or done juice fasting of any kind. I would suggest that you read <u>Volume 3</u> of this series titled, **"How to Lose 30 Pounds (Or More) In 30 Days With Juice Fasting."** There, I go step-by-step through the recipe, the juicing process and basically lay it all out in detail.

Nonetheless, if you want to get started right away and do not necessarily want to spend the time juicing any fruits or veggies, then do this: Go to the supermarket and purchase the freshest kind of fruit and veggie juice that you can find. When I say 'freshest,' I mean NOT from concentrate, powdered or any other of those sugar-infested brands.

When I say fruit juice, I do NOT mean Kook-Aid. Find juices that are natural and have no sugar added. Since you will be drinking these juices fairly quickly, opt for freshly squeezed if you can find them. As an alternative, I like the **Bolthouse Farms** brand. I use it sometimes when I do short fasts of one-to-three days and don't have time to juice or purchase fruits and veggies. This brand, however, does tend to have a lot of sugar. Therefore, it is highly recommended that you always **combine fruit and vegetable juice in a jar and then add water until the excessive sweetness is reduced.** If you are new to juice fasting, the key is to: **KEEP IT SIMPLE**.

You want to find a fruit/veggie juice combination that you enjoy. However, it may take a few tries before you find the right one for you. What matters most right now is that you <u>take action</u> and start working on your (**IF**) program so that you can reach your weight loss goals. You will discover the perfect fruit/veggie combination in the measure that you walk forward and get involved in the process.

How Much Juice Do I Drink?

If you decide to use juice fasting as your (**IF**) method, then it is important that you do not exceed 64 ounces of juice per day. As guidance, drink **an eight-to-twelve-ounce glass of juice every four hours**. The best way to structure the juice-drinking is to mix it in a one-gallon jug with a tight lid. Fill a cooler halfway with ice and then lay the jug down, making sure that the lid is tight. With a few plastic cups in the cooler, you can take it with you wherever you go and have your swig every four hours. The juice is your lifeline while you're fasting. So it is of great importance that you take it with you wherever you go.

Once you arrive at your destination, you can either keep it in the cooler (keep the cooler at hand), or you can refrigerate it.

One Gallon of Water Daily

No matter whether you are juice or water fasting, it is important that you drink at least one gallon of water daily. The water will help to fight off the hunger pangs and will also hydrate the body and aid in the detoxification process. It is very important that you drink the very best quality of water that you can. I know that tap water is usually good in most places, but I still would opt for filtered water - regardless. If you have a filter in your house, then that is the way to go.

If, however, tap water is the only kind that you have readily-available right now, then make it a point to boil it for like five minutes. I want you to drink absolutely pure, fresh water with ZERO chemicals or other toxins. Otherwise we are defeating the very purpose that you are fasting. Moreover, you may also wish to purchase some bottled water so that you can take a few with you when you're out.

One gallon of water daily is the recipe.

I cannot recommend a dry fast. If what you are feeling in your heart is that you need to do a dry fast, then that is something that you must settle within your own conscience. When I did my three-day dry fast, it was a very personal adventure that I undertook because I wanted to pass along the information to others. **But it is a very dangerous practice and should not be done lightly under any circumstances**. Best if done with the direct supervision of a medical professional. Take a moment and evaluate the various options we've just looked at. Which type of fast have you decided to do? Write about your decision in your fasting journal.

Additional Fasting Supplies

There are also a few other supplies that you can get **to help with the hunger and other symptoms**. To give you energy, try a cup of decaffeinated green tea in the afternoons (*or whenever weakness and hunger hit you the hardest*). During the day, when hunger comes, you can counterattack with a bottle of seltzer water (*sparkling* *water/club soda*). At night, to help you settle down and go to sleep, you can have a cup of chamomile tea. To sweeten the tea, use Stevia. Stay away from artificial sweeteners as Equal or Splenda. To help with hunger and detox symptoms, use decaffeinated green tea, chamomile tea and seltzer water (*sparkling water/club soda*). These tools will go a long ways to calm you whenever there's any type of physical, mental or emotional disturbance.

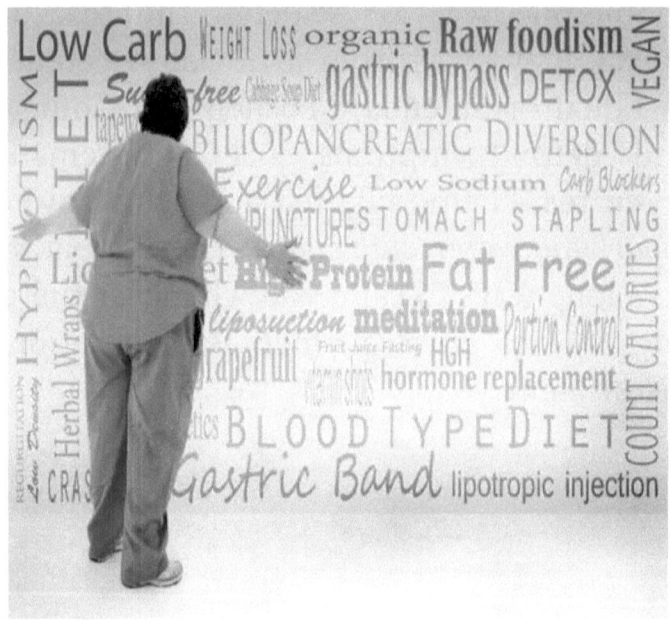

"One of the things that first attracted me to fasting is that it is very straightforward. I do not have to get sucked into the world of diets out there, which has always been very confusing and discouraging to me."

Chapter 5
How Fasting Works

One of the things that first attracted me to fasting is that it is very straightforward. If I am juice fasting, then I drink only juice and water. If I am water fasting, then I drink only water. And the weight loss and detox cleansing results are always tremendous. I do not have to get sucked into the crazy world of diets out there, which has always been very confusing and discouraging to me. Fasting was the way out and my personal fountain of youth and health. So, in this chapter, I want to talk about the process that fasting kicks into motion, and how the body respond when calories are restricted. The amazing process that I am referring to is known as **ketosis**.

Ketosis is the word used to describe the body's reaction to calorie-limitation. When in ketosis, the body is no longer receiving energy from food intake. Therefore, as a survival mechanism, it starts to get its fuel by devouring stored fat deposits. This process of Ketosis normally starts after approximately 16 hours of not eating. Since a lot of the worst toxins in your bodies accumulate in fat deposits, a temporary sickness ensues called a Healing Crisis (*or Curative Crisis.*). A little later we will look at the detox symptoms that one can expect to experience while fasting. All in all, this healing crisis is a very positive symptom. It won't feel like something good, but it means that all of that toxic filth in your body is being cleansed and expelled through the skin (sweating), feces and urine. The healing crisis usually lasts 9-11 days or until the body completely rids itself of all toxins.

Once the healing crisis has passed, most people begin to feel much more alert and energized. Once I pass 11 to 14 days of fasting, I normally feel like I can go on fasting indefinitely. **This is the most pleasant part of the fast**. I like to use the analogy of a man trapped in a brick room with no water. He knows that the water is in the next room, so he starts to pound on the wall with a hammer (*fasting*). Eventually (*after the discomfort and exertion*), the wall finally collapses and he is able to drink water and be refreshed. Fasting, to me, is like the breaking of an 'inner wall' that leads to great joy, peace and satisfaction. I hope that you get to experience this because there is really nothing like it.

As I said at the start of this book, what matters most is that you remain willing to take action to the very best of your ability. If you do that, I am certain that - sooner or later - you will experience the breakthrough that I have just described.

How Long Can I Water Fast?

This is a very common question. The best answer is: It depends on your body weight and amount of body fat. Basically, you can water fast for as long as the body has fat to eat. Once the amount of body fat is depleted, then you would go into 'real' starvation - also known as 'the second hunger.' While today it is typical to hear people say "*I am starving,*" I really don't think many know what starving really is (*and that's a blessing*). As I said earlier, after 9-11 days of water fasting (*once the body has detoxified*), hunger (*for many people*) becomes minimum and they feel they could go on for an indefinite period. Hunger returns (*violently*) when all of the body-fat has been consumed. At this point, real starvation sets in and the body begins to basically eat itself alive.

My 'Second Hunger' Experience

In one of my first extended water fasts, I experienced this second hunger for myself. It was a horrific and very painful experience. It literally felt as though there was an animal with fangs on my insides chewing and eating my organs and intestines. I could not help but weep deeply. I was able to end the fast with some grape juice and move towards restoring my body. But what of those (*children*) who are - right now - starving FOR REAL and have no way of immediately ending such terrible pain?

I experienced the excruciating pain but for a few hours. Many are experiencing it indefinitely. I'm telling you, that experience really hit home for me. It made me very grateful for everything that I have. I vowed never to complain anymore about anything in my life, no matter how upsetting.

Even if everything went wrong in my life from then on, it would NEVER, ever come close to the horror that many others are going through because they don't have enough to eat. Food for thought, huh? In short, I would tell you that the majority of people (*of average weight and good health*) can fast for around 40 days. t and has now begun to feed on live tissue. This is the start of real starvation. The fast **MUST** be broken at once. I experienced this *'second hunger'* years ago when I first started to practice water fasting. It was a very scary experience as I literally felt my skin and muscles being chewed from the inside out. That was my own carelessness. Fasting should <u>never</u> get to that phase.

For How Long Can I Juice Fast?

This is a question that I am getting more and more recently. As the huge health and weight loss benefits of juice fasting are discovered, more people are looking to this practice to solve their weight problem. And for those who are more than 50 pounds overweight, that usually translates to a long juice fast 60 days and above. Is this healthy?

The answer is: It depends on what ingredients are used. I could <u>NOT</u> endorse a juice fast of that length if it was comprised <u>only</u> of fruits and vegetables. And the reason is because fruits and vegetables have lots of nutrients but not very much (*if any*) protein, which the body needs. I have gotten into debates with friends in the medical field who say that the body should NEVER go without protein, even for a few days. Most of them, sadly, are flat-out against fasting. So nothing that I say makes them budge in any direction. I have even laid out scientific studies about the benefits of fasting. And not even that can sway their closed minds. At any rate, in relation to protein while fasting, I have learned that the body will find protein sources to consume via a process called 'catabolism.'

Catabolism is a very complex process with a lot of variables. For our purposes, however, it means that the body starts to eat some of the muscle tissue along with the fat deposits, meaning that some protein (*from the muscle tissue*) is being consumed and reabsorbed. I won't bore you with detailed scientific terminology, but the various alternative medicine PHD's that I've spoken to tell me that, thanks to catabolism, the body could go a few months without the direct consumption of protein. To be safe, however, I'd say one shouldn't juice fast for more than 60 days without introducing protein into the mix.

Juice Fasting & Protein

For anyone planning to do a juice fast longer than 60 days, it is important to add protein sources into the mix. I did a 100-day juice fast years ago and it was a very rewarding experience. I did not do it for weight loss per se, yet ended up losing 105 pounds. A juice fast of this length should include some protein via the mixture of crushed nuts, oils, tofu or spirulina, the amazing micro salt water plant that contains rich amounts of vegetable protein.

If a long juice fast includes these additional (*and necessary*) ingredients, one could possibly continue juice fasting indefinitely. This, however, is not common. The longest juice fasts that are normally carried out range from 30 to 60 days.

And, honestly... 30 days of juice fasting is more than enough to start. You can always fast again later for a longer period of time once you get used to the practice and get to know how your body responds with long-term calorie restriction.

Eating After Fasting

This is where the majority of people fall off the wagon and undo all of their hard work. I know that I said this before, but I must emphasize that: THE MOST **IMPORTANT PART OF ANY FAST IS WHAT YOU EAT AFTER THE FAST**. If you have read some of my other books, you know that I tend to be a bit of a pest repeating that over and over. But I want nothing but the very best for you. And I have seen just what happens when a person breaks a fast inappropriately. One man that I know fasted for 14 days with just water and broke it with a cheeseburger.

He ended up in the hospital with severe stomach inflammation. His belly almost tore and caused his death, although he recovered after ten days of great pain and suffering. Others fast for long periods of time, sacrificing their time and enduring hunger and detox symptoms to lose large amounts of weight. However, a few months later they have gained all of the weight back and are bitter, demoralized and depressed. That happened to me when I first started out and I can tell you that it was one of the most painful experiences that I've ever been through. The problem is that, a lot of attention is given to the fasting, but very little (if any) is given to the process of breaking the fast. You can lose a tremendous amount of weight with intermittent fasting (IF). But if you do nothing more... if you have not planned ahead as to what your diet will be when the fast ends, then you are setting yourself up for failure. **Let me be blunt**: *Nothing sucks as bad as fasting for 30 days, going through the hunger, detox and sacrifice to lose weight, only to see yourself balloon right back up in a few short weeks after the fast because you didn't change your eating habits.*

And I can guarantee you that, if you do not change your eating habits, then chances are **VERY** high that you **WILL** regain the weight you lose by fasting within three months. I need you to be very aware of this reality now when we are just getting started. Ponder on what I've just said as we move forward. I will give you. However, **YOU** are the one that has to be convinced. **Here's the bottom line**: fasting for weight loss without a plan for permanent eating-habit changes is like spitting up in the air. You will **NOT** be happy at all.

Chapter 6
Cleaning Up Your Act

One of the most important steps to take prior to starting any **(IF)** program is to cleanup your act. In other words, cut out the junk in your diet 7-10 days before starting to fast. I have found this to be very effective because it will help the body **begin the weight loss and detox process in advance**. In addition, junk foods are the ones that we get most addicted to and cause the <u>strongest withdrawal cravings</u>. Getting them out of the picture right away will help to reduce the force of the hunger and cravings when you start fasting later because some of those toxins will have already been eliminated.

Besides, giving up junk food sends a signal to your mind loud and clear that this is <u>not</u> going to be a temporary path. Instead, I want your **(IF)** efforts to be part of a permanent change in your overall diet and health. For at least 10 days prior to starting any intermittent fasting structure, cut out the foods listed below from your diet. In fact, cut them out completely - <u>whether or not you're fasting</u>. A lot of these foods may have a strong hold on you. Letting them go in itself will be a big accomplishment. Trust me. Following these directions will give you huge (*and very fast*) results. It may be uncomfortable at the beginning, but you will get used to it. **And you'll be very happy when you see the pounds start to melt off of your body.** Let's take a look at the foods that I want you to eliminate from your diet:

Banned Foods

(Avoid at all times, regardless of whether you're fasting or not)

*Salt

* Sugar

* Fried Foods

* Cheese

* Dairy Products

* Red Meat

* Alcohol

* Butter or Margarine

* Fruit Juices (Except the ones you may use for juice fasting, of course)

* Regular Ketchup (except low sodium)

*Junk Food of ANY Kind (cheeseburgers, pizza, donuts, pastries, cakes, candy etc...)

The Salt Factor

Cutting out salt was one of the steps which helped me to lose lots of weight quickly, especially in the first few weeks. When we are overweight, a lot of the weight is from water retained due to the excessive consumption of sodium. If you take a look at most of the canned and pre-packaged products sold in supermarkets, the majority of them are packed with sodium. Take a look and you'll see what I mean. All of that excess sodium doesn't do the body any good and it certainly doesn't help the weight loss process much either.

The key is to give the body 'adequate' amounts of sodium. That can be done by eating **PROPERLY**. The list of foods that I have given you above all have plenty of natural sodium. In the majority of cases, adding salt to what we eat is simply not necessary. In fact, I no longer add salt to anything. At first it was hard because I had become so accustomed to eating very salty. Today, however, I do not add any salt to the food that I eat. If you look at the shopping list I have provided below, you will see that I have listed plenty of 'no salt' seasoning options. So the point isn't to eat bland food that tastes like cardboard. The point is to remove that which is excessive and that the body can acquire naturally from a <u>clean diet</u>.

Foods to Limit
(When You Aren't Fasting)

*Fruits (Stick To Strawberries or Cantaloupe)
* Tomatoes
* Peas or Corn
* Olive Oil

The Sugar Monster

This is the biggie. Most people who are overweight are <u>hopelessly</u> addicted to sugar. I know that I was. I was amazed to learn that <u>refined sugar is actually toxic to the body.</u> If you have ever overindulged in refined sugar and woken up the following morning feeling like a zombie, then you know exactly what I'm talking about. Refined sugar gives us a short-term shot of energy. However, the energy surge quickly results in a *'crash.'* The crash is evident by the ongoing craving for more and more sugar. For people who eat a lot of sugar, these cravings can be very strong - nearly blinding. Sugar gives us that little bit of energy, but it promptly takes it away and - soon - we are back to square one - zapped. We never receive the substantial, healthy and lasting energy that we get through complex carbohydrates and lean proteins. So, if you are a sugar addict as I was, I implore you with all that is in me to fight, fight... fight to overcome this destructive monster. If you do that alone, you will take large strides toward measurable weight loss and health improvement.

I was stuck in sugar addiction for many years. Every time that the cravings hit me, I gave in by eating more refined sugar. The first time that I started to resist, the detox symptoms were very so strong that I almost passed out. I felt like someone coming off hard drugs like cocaine or heroin. Such is the destructive power of refined sugar. Even though it was hard, about 72 hour later, when the sugar was totally out of my body, I started to feel a sense of tranquility and wellbeing that is indescribable. The cravings were greatly reduced. I realized that the worst was over. As long as I did not fall back into its grasp, I was free of the sugar monster. It was a great feeling and, if sugar is a problem for you, I hope that you, too, get a chance to experience that same freedom.

My point is this: No matter what the short-term discomfort may be, letting go of refined sugars is **the very best thing I have ever done for my physical and mental health**. I say *'mental health'* because sugar caused me to always be in a state of confusion, depression and anxiety that curtailed my ability to function. In addition, I kept waking up in the middle of the night craving more, more and more sugar, so I was not even sleeping well. Can you relate to any of these symptoms? **Do not compare**. Identify. Even if the symptoms you experience *'aren't as severe,'* as the ones that I did, you still will do yourself a huge favor by eliminating refined sugar. This is the beginning of the process. For now, continue to eat whatever else you have been eating **EXCEPT** for the banned foods. Below is a sample of the shopping list that I return to when I am not fasting.

Shopping List

*Boneless Chicken Breast

*Extra Lean Ground Turkey Breast (*no deli turkey*)

*Egg Whites

Note: I use the liquid egg whites that come in a box because all I have to do is toss them in the pan. Besides, I always make a huge mess separating the yolk! :-)

*Low Sodium Tuna Fish

Note: This kind usually can be found in envelopes rather than cans.

*Fresh Fish (*Tilapia and Grouper. Salmon Once Weekly ONLY*)

*Baked Potatoes

*Sweet Potatoes

*Quaker Oats (*100% Whole Grain, Quick Oats*)

*Cream of Wheat (*White Box*)

*Cream of Rice

*Pasta (*Only Whole Grain or Whole Wheat - No Egg Noodles*)

*Brown Rice

Note: I am lazy and use the boil-in-the-bag rice.

*Fresh Green Vegetables (*Broccoli, Carrots, Cauliflower etc...*)

Note: These are great for steaming. I usually purchase the bags that come with them already pre-mixed. You will find a lot of different veggie combinations to choose from in these pre-mixed bag selections. I like these because all I have to do is wash them and steam them.

*Balsamic Vinegar

*Garlic Powder

*Onion Powder

*Enricos No Salt-No Fat Spaghetti Sauce (*Or Any Other No-Salt Brand You Find*)

Note: This Enricos brand may be hard to find. Check out the 'health food' area in your supermarket or a separate shelf in the pasta aisle with the healthy pastas and sauces.

*Stevia Sweetener (*No Equal or Splenda*)

Note: Stevia is a leaf and is not piled with all of the chemical trash they put in other artificial sweeteners. It does have a bit of an aftertaste, but you will get used to it after a while. :-)

*Any Sugar-Free and Low-Sodium Salad Dressing

Note: It may take a few minutes to find the right salad dressing that meets these parameters. Ask the supermarket clerk for assistance

if you are unable to see anything in the shelves. My personal favorite is the Olde Cape Cod Raspberry Light dressing.
*Mrs. Dash No Salt All-Purpose Seasoning

If you end your periods of intermittent fasting by returning to a diet based on this shopping list, **AND** you also work at staying away from the banned foods, I can tell you with certainty (*based on personal experience*) that you will start to lose A LOT of weight quickly. Better yet, you will KEEP IT OFF.

Chapter 7
Setting a Foundation

At this point, there are a couple of questions that I want you to write and answer in your journal. One of the reasons why people start a weight loss program and fall off is because, when hit by temptation, they are - at that moment - unable to remember with sufficient power the important reasons why they want to lose weight in the first place. Blinded by hunger, detox symptoms and other types of temptation, they give in and eat what they shouldn't. The enjoyment, however, is very short-lived as, almost immediately, the **Three Horsemen of Guilt, Shame and Accusation** arrive and start tormenting the person. If you have ever started a weight loss program and quit halfway through, then I am pretty sure that you know what I'm talking about. The result of this emotional onslaught is that the person often will say *"screw it"* and abandon the diet altogether. *"What's the use? I'm a weakling, a loser... I will never lose all of this weight! Why even try? This is pointless. I'm hopeless!"*

Many people are stuck in this demoralizing trap of falling, giving up, gaining weight and then starting the diet again weeks, months (*or years*) later. I can't think of anything that is more frustrating that this. Well, **the questions that I want you to answer here are designed to erect a fortress against these temptations**. Here's my point: If you can overcome the temptation directly when it hits, then you will not put the wrong food in your mouth and start the entire compulsive episode. That's what we want. To stop the *'screw it'* syndrome BEFORE it has a chance to take hold.

Many people tell me: *"Robert if I hadn't eaten that fifth donut, I would be fine."* I always try to help them understand: *"It isn't the fifth donut that gets you, it's the first one! If you don't eat the first one, then you certainly won't eat the second, third, fourth or fifth. It is the FIRST one that starts all of the trouble. And it is the first one that we must learn to avoid."* Does that make sense? So, right now, I want you to take some time and **write the questions listed below in your journal and then answer them with as much honesty as you can muster**. Don't just skimp over them. Take your time and answer them thoroughly and in detail.

The answers that you come up with represent the artillery that you will use when temptation invites you to stray from your diet. At that particular moment of temptation, all that will be between you and that piece of junk food will be the answers that you write to these questions. So here we go:

What will happen short-term if I DO NOT resist these urges and continue down the same road? In other words, over the coming days, weeks and months, how is your life going to be and how are you going to feel if you do nothing and allow these habits to go on unbridled? Be as explicit as you can.

(Example: If I do nothing and fail to resist these urges, I will continue to gain weight and feel worse and worse about myself. I will isolate because I'll feel ashamed of my appearance. I won't want to be seen, go out in public. I will be depressed and feel defeated etc...")

What is the ultimate long-term consequence that I will pay if I do not take action NOW to change these thinking and behavior patterns as they

relate to food and eating? Be explicit!

(Example: If I do not take action now and do whatever it takes to lose this weight, I will feel like I failed at something that is very important to me, I won't have the same self-esteem because I'll continue to be fat. I will feel defeated and absolutely terrible because there is nothing that I want more than to get rid of this excess weight and look and feel my best etc...)

What will my life be like in 10 years if I do not take action now? Mentally, physically, socially, spiritually etc... Remember *The Ghost of Christmas Future from A Christmas Carroll*? Well, this is it. Use it! Dig deep into your heart and mind and look at yourself 10, 15 years from now **NOT** having done anything about your weight and health. What do you see? How do you look? How do you feel? How is your health? How is your quality of life?

(Example: Ten years from now I look like a beached whale plumped in the sofa with dark circles around my eyes, no energy to do anything and in deep depression and isolation because I am disgusted with my appearance and have withdrawn from life

completely. I am sitting there wishing I was dead etc..")

Am I willing to pay these negative consequences? Why not? Be detailed. *(Example: because I want to be around for my children, travel abroad, get married, continue to advance in my career, be prosperous, have a lavish life, not develop a chronic illness etc).* As I said earlier, it is important that you take your time and come up with strong answers. If you just jot down a one-sentence response without giving the questions deep and serious thought, then you are wasting your time.

(Example: I am NOT willing to pay these horrible consequences. I am prepared to do ANYTHING to keep that horrible future from ever coming to pass. That means that I am now willing and prepared to resist any hunger and any temptation so that I can overcome this weight issue once and for all and avoid having to face a future that is so ugly and hopeless etc...)

These questions are meant to strip your soul bear and **force you to cough up deep-seated thoughts and feelings**. That is not to say that initially you may only come up with one sentence. That is fine. But don't give up... keep meditating on the question and continue to probe your mind and heart for answers. Believe me, they are there!

How would I feel if I STOPPED feeding into these food impulses and began to say said NO? (*Example: Empowered, Good about myself, Hopeful etc*). Why would I feel these positive feelings? (*Example: Because I will have resisted something that harms me, because I will have gained self-esteem, because I would start to feel lighter, healthier, more attractive etc*).

This is the pivotal point where you can begin to see that <u>NOT</u> giving in to these urges is the <u>ONLY</u> way to true happiness and satisfaction. Giving in may feel good at that immediate moment, but saying no and delaying gratification is the road to the ultimate victory that you seek.

What would happen if I resist these urges to eat? Do I feel like I would collapse or die? Can I recognize that these are lies? Explain the reasons the mind gives you as to why resisting these food impulses is 'too hard' or even 'impossible.'

(Example: When I am tempted, I feel like I simply cannot resist. The cravings are just too strong). Can you internalize the reality that this is a lie? That you are **NOT** helpless? That you **CAN** get through it?

(Example: Resisting these cravings is NOT impossible because I will NOT die if I do not give in, etc). The key to this question is realizing that any short-term discomfort you may feel from resisting the food urges will pass, that you will not fall to pieces if you hold your ground.

As a matter of fact, I can tell you from firm experience that cravings and temptations rarely last more than 30 minutes. Once they pass, the sense of satisfaction is amazing.

What is the ultimate truth for you?

(Example: I must change my impulsive eating and I must stop giving in to the cravings and food urges because otherwise I will never reach my goal, I will feel unhappy, I will feel unfulfilled, I risk illness etc). In view of the answers to all of the previous questions, what conclusion have you reached?

So, to round up, **what real choice do you have than to change?** Continuing to give in to hunger through binging, nibbling and/or compulsive eating is not the answer. It will never be the answer. It will never work. *Continuing to give in to binging, nibbling and/or compulsive overeating will always lead you to negative outcomes in your life.* Period. End of story!

Can you admit this to yourself and understand it? Explain why you admit it and why you understand it. If you can admit to yourself that the status-quo doesn't work and that immediate change is imperative, and if you can write here in detail the reasons why this is so, then you are on your way to some pretty dramatic changes in your food behaviors.

So this begs the question: **What is your choice going to be?**

(Example: My choice will be to do whatever it takes and go through whatever short-term discomfort I need to in order to overcome and reach my weight loss goals). Explain the "why" of your choice.

What are you willing to do to achieve the life that you deserve? Here we reinforce the previous question with detail of what you are now prepared to do to reach your goals.

(Example: I am willing to walk through the urge to binge, feel the pain of not doing so, deal with hunger pains directly even if I want to give up and give in) This last answer is important because it provides powerful reasons for you to hang on to when you feel like giving up. So be detailed!

If you follow my instructions and answer the above questions thoroughly and with total honesty, you will have created a <u>very powerful weapon</u> against that 'first bite' of food that knocks you off your diet, fast etc...

Here's how you are going to use these questions: When you start fasting and find yourself hit with hunger, detox symptoms and/or any kind of emotional negativity that make you want to quit, take out your journal and start reading the questions one-by-one. At that particular moment, try to add more to each one of the answers as you go through them.

Focus all of your attention on reading the questions, answers and adding to them. **Give yourself totally to this task**. In my experience, after 10 or 15 minutes, I am re-energized and get a fresh jolt of motivation to continue. The answer of 'how will I feel in 10 years if I don't take action' is the one that always gets me. The vision of myself ten years into the future still obese and having done nothing filled me with such fear and disgust that I literally didn't care how hungry or weak I got. All I cared about was reaching my goal.

While fasting, you will also want to be in touch with other people that are on the same road. To that end, I have put together **TWO** fasting forums, which you can access by visiting the main website FitnessThroughFasting.com. There are lots of people there who are ready and willing to motivate and encourage you as you walk through your fast. And there are lots of folks there who can use your support as well. You will be surprised how hunger and detox symptoms often vanish when you focus on giving motivation to somebody else who needs it. Give and you shall receive!

Chapter 8
Lose 15 Pounds (Or More) Every Month

By this point you should be very clear as to what type of fasting you wish to do, whether water, juice or perhaps a combination of both. You have received a list of banned foods which, as instructed, should be removed from your diet at least 10 days before you start fasting.

I've also given you a partial shopping list that shows you the kind of diet that you should consider following when you're not fasting. Moreover, we have worked on a series of questions designed to give you that extra shot of motivation whenever temptation threatens to knock you off your course.

You have answered the questions honestly and thoroughly in your fasting journal and have visited various online forums, registered and introduced yourself. You have covered a lot of ground, been diligent in your preparation and are now ready to jump into (**IF**).

Let's take a look at what I call the **5 (IF) Methods For Ultimate Weight Loss & Health.** I want you to read through this entire section and, in the end, choose which one of these (IF) methods you feel most comfortable with. Later, I will walk you a day of fasting with general tips and steps you can follow to get through hunger and other symptoms. Over time, I want you to try <u>ALL</u> of these five methods, get good at them and use them interchangeably. Done consistently, intermittent fasting can help you to lose 15 pounds (*or more*) every month. The key is to break the fast each time with clean food and **NOT** indulge in any of the '<u>banned foods</u>.' Do that, and you <u>WILL</u> lose lots of weight quickly. I have seen it happen in my own life and with many others.

Daily Intermittent Fasting: As in Catholic Lent Fasting and Muslim Ramadan, here you fast from sunup to sundown - <u>approximately 12 hours daily</u>. The fast is broken each night with a light meal in compliance with the banned foods and shopping list I gave you earlier. The meals that you eat at night must be light and clean. You get to eat every night, so that in itself should serve as comfort to the mind that is always obsessing about food. Your *"eating window"* remains open until dawn, but for most of that time you will be sleeping. If you are a raw beginner, have a lot of weight to lose and/or have eaten poorly for many years, you can scale down **Daily (IF)** and start reducing the number of hours per day during which you do not eat. In other words, instead of <u>NOT</u> eating for 12 hours, cut the fasting window to eight or six.

What is your usual eating schedule? What is the longest amount of time that you normally go through daily without eating? Whatever it is, double it. If you normally eat every four hours, then start by extending it to 8 hours, and so on. Do that until you are able to complete the full 12 hours of fasting in one day. That is a very good way to start getting used to calorie restriction. <u>My point is this</u>: There is no race. If at first all you can do is six or eight hours of intermittent fasting, then that is great.

Remember what I said at the start of this book: What matters most is your willingness to do this to the very best of your ability. Progress, not perfection, is the key.

Twelve hours to eat, twelve hours to fast... and so the cycle continues each day.

You can get up in the AM, have breakfast, and then fast for the next 12 hours. I love **Daily (IF)**. It is great for beginners and the experienced alike. After a few days, many like to add hours to the daily fast as they are motivated. For example, on a particular day, one may eat at night but decide to skip breakfast or vice versa. Experienced folks use this kind of **(IF)** indefinitely. I know one person who fasted daily in this fashion for five years! Amazing..

Estimated Weekly weight loss: three to five pounds. With this type of **(IF)**, you can lose 15 pounds every month (*or more*).

Some people have written me to say that they lost 25-30 pounds in only **ONE** month, using **Daily (IF)**. It is a simple system, but very powerful. Giving the body 12 hours daily of fasting does amazing things, not only weight loss but overall cleansing, tissue repair and detoxification.

Every-Other-Day Intermittent Fasting:
Another form of intermittent fasting is to go
for an entire 24-hour cycle every other day.
Example: You fast from 8am Monday
morning to 8am Tuesday morning. Eat
lightly on Tuesday. Wake up on Wednesday
at 7:30am and have breakfast. Start the fast
at 8am until the same time on Thursday...
and so on. Estimated Weekly weight loss:
two to four pounds.

Half-Week Intermittent Fasting: Fast for
3.5 days of the week. Example: Fast from
8am Monday to 8pm Thursday. You can
return to regular eating for the rest of the
week. **Fasting would resume the
following Monday at 8am - repeating the
same cycle.** This system requires caution,
however. Since one does not eat for 84-hour
periods, it will be necessary to follow the
breaking a fast instructions, listed towards
the end of this book. Estimated weekly
weight loss: three to five pounds.

Seven-Day Intermittent Fasting: Fast for
an entire seven days, return to your regular
diet for seven days, and then fast for another
seven days. Similar to the Half Week
method, you will need follow the breaking a

fast instructions. Estimated weekly weight loss: Five to 20 pounds during initial 7-day fast and five to seven on subsequent ones.

Combination Intermittent Fasting: The ultimate way to practice intermittent fasting is to combine all of the above and complete 14 and 30-day cycles of intermittent fasts. Combination can also be doing 24-hour juice fasting once a week, three-day juice fasting weekly or bi-weekly... whatever is within your ability to do, **THAT** is more than enough to get started. Combination (**IF**) is my very favorite because it units the previous four (IF) methods into 14 and 30-day cycles of intermittent fasts.

Here's how it works:

• Start, for example, on a Monday by doing **Daily (IF) for THREE DAYS**. When you break the fast on Wednesday evening, keep the *"eating-window"* open for 12 hours as usual.

• On Thursday morning, jump to **Every Other Day (IF)** and carry out a 24-hour fast. Break the fast on Friday morning and keep the *"eating-window"* open for 24 hours.
• Launch another **24-hour fast** on Saturday

morning and break it on Sunday when you wake up. You are done for the week. Following this structure, **you will have fasted 84 hours in seven days (3.5 days).**

• On Monday, you can move forward and carry out the **Half Week (IF)** system. Basically, you will fast all day and night Monday, Tuesday and Wednesday – breaking the fast on Thursday evening. Go back to eating for the rest of the week, always paying attention to keeping a clean diet that steers clear of items in the banned foods list.

Having done this **Half-Week (IF)**, you will have fasted for another 84 hours (3.5 *days*) and, altogether, completed 7 days of intermittent fasting spread out over two weeks. Want to keep going? Do it!

•To finish the month strong, continue on week three with **Seven Day (IF)**. Here you fast round-the-clock for an entire week *(Monday morning to Sunday morning)*, totaling 168 solid hours of fasting (7 days). This is **TWICE** what you did in weeks one and two.   Return to eating on Sunday morning (follow the breaking a fast instructions below).

Following this **Combination (IF)** structure, by month's end, <u>you will have completed 14 solid days of fasting spread out over a four-week period</u>. **TWO WHOLE WEEKS OF FASTING!** Amazing! And this is just **ONE** example of how you can combine the different **(IF)** structures.

I am sure that, if you get creative, you can come up with many more options. And the results are astounding! I have received letters from readers who said they carried out **Combination (IF)** to the letter for an entire month and have seen remarkable results.

One person did **Every Other Day (IF)** for 30 days and lost 50 pounds! As I said already, what matters is that you jump aboard and get going. **By no means pressure yourself to do a long fast that you aren't mentally prepared to do**. A lot of people that have fasted for 14 days and beyond first had to begin with shorter ones <u>to build their stamina</u>. So, if you are experienced and have done it before, then bon voyage - you're on your way. If, on the other hand, you are new to fasting, then do what you can. No matter what you are able to do, you come off a winner!

Chapter 9
Launching The Fast

•Once you have chosen which type of (**IF**) plan you are going to follow, pick a start day! Open your fasting journal and record the day. I suggest that you start as soon as possible, over the next few days. Keep the momentum. If you procrastinate and let time go by, the effect is not the same. The mind is tricky and will try to convince you to put it off indefinitely. So please don't let this lag!

•Go shopping and make sure that you have lots of clean food in the house. Stock up on drinking water, seltzer/sparkling water, green tea and chamomile tea. As I mentioned earlier, seltzer water is great to soothe hunger pangs and detox symptoms, green tea will give you a pep of energy when you feel weak, and chamomile tea is great to drink at nights to settle the belly and help you fall asleep.

You may want to also pick up a bottle of Tryptophan 500mg tablets. Tryptophan is an amino acid that will help stabilize your mood when hunger and detox symptoms hit, and it also can help you to sleep if the chamomile isn't enough. If you cannot find tryptophan, you can opt for Valerian Root capsules instead for sleep support and as a calming agent.

•Plan your meals for the days in between the fasting. This, of course, would not apply if you chose the 7-day plan since once done you would simply return to eating for a full seven days. Otherwise, make sure to **KNOW** ahead of time what you are going to eat on those "*days off*"! Use the sample menu that I gave you earlier and stock up on healthy foods. Make sure that all foods on the banned list are **OUT** of the house - good riddance.

IF, you live with children or (for some other reason), you simply cannot get rid of all goodies - then ask your spouse to 'hide them' or put them somewhere where you will not be able to access them easily. Of course this won't work with refrigerated food, but you can maximize your 'security zone' by making sure that the majority of the tempting food is out of sight.

•Go to Fasting Forum I and/or Fasting Forum II at **FitnessThroughFasting.com**, bookmark the pages and plan on spending time reading and posting messages **DAILY** while you are fasting. I started those forums for the exclusive purpose of bringing *"fasters"* together so that we could motivate and support one another. So use it! There are some amazing posts that will inspire and help you get through the rough spots. Don't do this alone!

• If you have not already done so, I want you to spend as much time as possible working on the nine 'foundation' questions that we discussed earlier. Answering those questions thoroughly and honestly will keep you busy, as well as motivate and encourage you by clarifying your values, dreams and goals.

The Day of The Fast

• Eat your last meal no later than 10Pm the previous night. If you wake up in the middle of the night hungry, drink a large glass of water and go back to bed. Upon awakening, drink two large glasses of water and make yourself a cup of green tea. If you are accustomed to doing morning devotionals, go ahead and do them. Drink your tea. Spend some time going over the foundation questions - keep adding to them. Remember: the answers are going to be your ammunition against hunger and the temptation to eat.

• Get used to visiting the online forums that I mentioned above. Read some of the posts. Pick a few that grab your attention and plan on posting replies later in the afternoon. Or, if you are so moved, go ahead and post a message right then and there. **Fasting Forum II** has a board specifically for fasting journals. You can either start your own journal or read about other people's fasting experiences. You'll find lots of powerful stuff there.

• If you have to leave your home to work or do errands, make sure to stock up on sparkling/seltzer water and tea. If you spend a lot of time in your car, purchase a small cooler and fill it with ice, water and seltzer. Carry a pack of sugarless gum with you. The act of chewing will distract you and calm hunger.

Water, seltzer and tea are your best friends while you are fasting. They are your allies. They fight on your behalf. They give you the edge you need to overcome detox symptoms and hunger pains. Learn to look at water, seltzer and tea as your "fasting tools". Always keep them close at hand.

• In the morning hours, drink a large glass of water anytime hunger strikes. Chew gum. But be careful: when hunger strikes, you will likely chew the gum with great fury and intensity. Take care not to bite your tongue! Ouch!

• One hour prior to your usual lunch time, open a bottle of sparkling/seltzer water and sip on it. The effervescence will settle the belly. Drink more water. Chew more gum.

• At lunch time, drink a tall glass of water and make yourself a cup of green tea. This is a good time to sit down and keep reading, studying and highlighting the answers in your journal. If you practice a religion, try having a time of prayer and petition. Open your fasting journal and write another entry; how are you feeling mentally and physically? Dump your thoughts and emotions on the journal. Write about your hopes and dreams. This will help you now and also in the future as you look back at it.

• The afternoon is usually the hardest time as one is prone to feel weakness, irritability and more intense hunger. **So drink lots of water!** Chew more gum! At around 3pm, prepare a cup of green tea. Please do not drink more than three cups per day. Green tea does contain some caffeine and, if drank in excess, can cause nervousness and anxiety. **OR**, purchase decaffeinated green tea instead.

• Drink more water. Open another bottle of seltzer/sparkling water. Chew more gum. Pray. Scream! Whatever it takes. Hang in there! The intense hunger peaks at around 4:30pm and normally becomes much more tolerable by 6pm. It, however, has a tendency to return at around 8pm – especially if your mind is idle. So stay busy!

• **NOW** is a good time to visit the fasting forums and post a message. Find a post from someone who is hurting and struggling. Believe me; the forums are filled with fellow fasters who are going through the same (*or worse*) difficulties as you. Write some words of comfort and support. Try doing that more than once. In fact, try comforting and motivating **THREE** fellow fasters. There is something extremely powerful in helping someone else while we ourselves are having difficulties. It always brings relief, not to mention that it takes the focus away from **ME** and puts it on the needs of another. Try it!

• In the evening, you can: spend time with your loved ones, drink more water, drink sparkling /seltzer water, read/write on the journal, watch TV, read a book, surf the Internet, go for a walk, chew gum, spend more time writing on your fasting journal, go to sleep... you name it. **I always make it a point to write a brief entry on the journal every night describing how the day went**. That is a good practice. Go to bed early. Sleeping will consume at least eight hours of fasting.

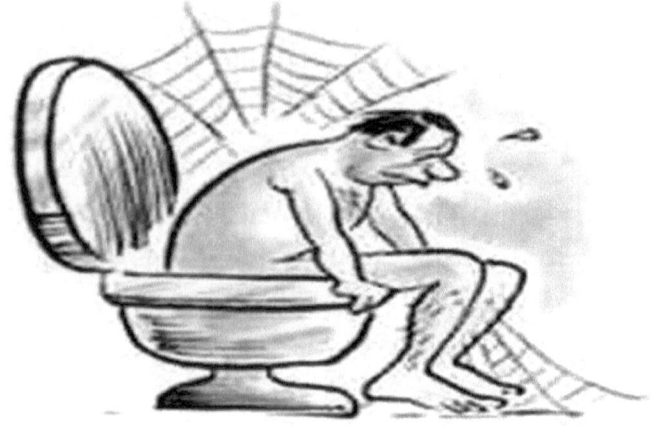

"A common fasting detox symptom is that all of the fecal matter adhered to your colon will either start gushing out in diarrhea or incite short-term constipation. The cobwebs are an exaggeration."

Chapter 10
Detox Symptoms

Here are some of the major symptoms that you may experience while you're fasting:

Headaches – This one is especially marked for coffee drinkers, but is also the case for persons who consume large amounts of sugar and alcohol. This symptom can really take a person out of commission. A lot of my colleagues call me a heretic for saying this, but if you need to take a couple of ibuprofen tablets to ease the pain, then so be it. Usually two tablets will do the trick. But don't take more than four daily. You may need to go through a little pain and discomfort. The good news is that headaches rarely last more than 72 hours, if that.

Dizziness – The body is not used to being deprived of eating whatever it wants and will go through dizzy spells, particularly during the first 11 days. The best solution for dizziness is to move slowly and get as much rest as your daily schedule allows.

Difficulty Performing Basic Tasks – Since with intermittent fasting you'll be eating notably less, it will take some time for the body to adjust, so you will more than likely feel very weak and may have trouble getting around in the first days. If you slow down and work on focusing on the individual tasks you are performing, this symptom can be overcome. It is important, however, for you to realize that **your body is going through a transition**. So you must move slowly and not try to push yourself too hard. You may not be able to function at the same capacity as you are accustomed. Fine. Slow down and give the body time to work on your behalf.

Weakness means that you need to be extra careful when walking around, and especially when getting up from a sitting position. Avoid harsh and/or abrupt movements. Move slowly, watch your step closely and always have something that you can hang on to if you suddenly feel like you are fainting. This is good advice. One time I totally hit the deck because I got up to quickly from a chair. I missed the corner of the wall by centimeters, but still hit myself quite hard on the floor.

This is about improving our health, not about getting hurt. Please be careful. I mean it. Be careful.

Pulsating Hunger Pains that disappear and then re-emerge throughout the day. For some persons, hunger is bad in the morning. But for the vast majority, the **hunger troll shows up <u>mostly at nig</u>**ht. Hunger will always be a part of our lives, and it is our task to master it rather than allow it to enslave us as it **<u>CAN AND WILL</u>** if we let it. In my case, hunger was very strong in my first three or four intermittent fasts. Then I found myself getting used to always being '*a little*' hungry. After a while, I loved it because I began to feel more alert, more energetic, optimistic...

I slept better. I actually **SLEPT THROUGH THE NIGHT** and woke up feeling terrific. Before the fast, I constantly woke up at night, usually like a raving lunatic wanting to raid the refrigerator. After a while, all of those terrible symptoms diminished and ultimately vanished. I would go to sleep at 11PM, close my eyes and, when I opened them, it was 6AM! For me, this was nothing less than a total miracle. And I felt great... refreshed and ready to go!

All of that just from getting used to eating less and being a little hungry. Much better than getting stuffed like a boar as I used to.

Bad Breath, Metallic Taste in Mouth, White Sticky Film on Tongue – These are all good indications that your body you body is eliminating toxicity. Most of these symptoms pass after nine-to-eleven days of fasting, or after a few weeks of ongoing intermittent fasts.

Bad Breath, I suggest that you get sugarless mints and keep them handy until the process ends.

Metallic Taste In the Mouth usually means that there are excessive (*and toxic*) heavy metals accumulated in your system. I recall during my first cleansing diet tasting constant sulfur and '*steel*' in my mouth for like one week.

White Sticky Film on the Tongue is completely repulsive but necessary. It's just another way for your body to get rid of all of the crap in your body that has kept you addicted to junk and overweight. For these symptoms, the best thing you can do is to keep drinking a lot of water.

Make sure to brush your teeth regularly. Keep a travel toothbrush with you if you spend a lot of time out. Mouthwash is also helpful.

Diarrhea or Constipation – All of the fecal matter adhered to your colon will either start gushing out in diarrhea or incite short-term constipation. I know that this is disgusting, but it happens. If you have eaten poorly for a long time, or have simply abused sugar or fat, your body may respond to this cleanse by starting to expel all of the toxic filth in this fashion.

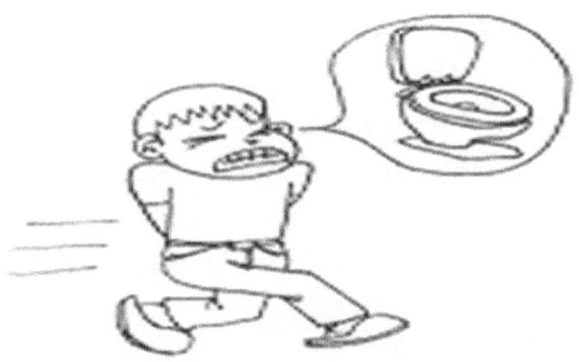

If Diarrhea Strikes, simply continue to follow the cleansing diet as outlined. Should it become severe, see your pharmacist and ask him or her for an over-the-counter recommendation. Continue with the fast.

The fasting process is a shock to the body, but it will finally get the message and react favorably to what you are doing. If you have diarrhea, make sure to keep yourself hydrated. Make it a point to drink at least one gallon of water daily. Stay close to a bathroom at all times. If you go out, make sure that you are always aware where the nearest restroom is. Seriously, you want to get to the toilet promptly anytime you need to.

If Constipation is The Case: visit your local pharmacy and ask your pharmacist about a stool softener. I personally use a herbal laxative called **Herbs & Prunes**. It works like a charm every time and is not harsh on my stomach. Take one tablet to start. Do not exceed four tablets in one day. But do this only if you fail to eliminate anything for at least three days. Give your body enough time to do it on its own.

Irritability / Mood Swings – If you have ever seen The Flintstones, you may remember Fred walking around growling on the episode where he is placed on a diet. Sooooo, be prepared to be a little *"short-fused"* during this time of heavy-duty preparation. Be aware that you will not be as patient as you normally would be. Tell your loved ones not to take it personally if - initially - you are less social that what they are accustomed. **This Is Normal & Will Pass!**

Facial Puffiness & Feeling Bloated – This symptom is much more marked for persons who consume large amounts of salt and/or sugar. The body is, in essence, disoriented when sugar and salt intake is so minimized and many times retains water for some days and becomes *"hyper-sensitive"* and toxic.

I personally was bloated to the max like the Stay Puft Marshmallow man. So being puffy was nothing new. It looked like somebody had stuck huge balloons on my cheeks. It was hideous. The cleansing diet took care of that and my face today is that of a normal human being rather than a cartoon character.

But these too will pass and are normal.

Note: Of course, if at any time you see that any of these symptoms continue and do not go away (*particularly after 11 days*), then you may have a more serious condition and should visit a medical practitioner at once.

It is certainly not my intention to tell you not to see your doctor or to neglect symptoms of what could be a more serious illness.

Chapter 11
Breaking The Fast

The sample schedule above should give you a general idea of how to get through each day of fasting. Since this is an intermittent fast, your instructions are to return to a clean diet on your days off. However, it is important that you break each fast properly. Here's how:

• If you chose **Daily (IF):** In this case you will only be fasting for roughly 12 hours daily. So breaking the fast is simple. Each night, break the fast with a vegetable (only a sprinkle of olive oil and salt) or fruit salad (sliced apples and pears, for example). Drink a large glass of water. Wait one hour. Then eat your dinner in strict observance of the guidelines I've already given you. In other words, eat clean and stay away from all of the banned foods. That's it!

• If you chose **Every Other Day (IF):** Break the fast with a vegetable or fruit salad. Wait **FOUR** hours, during which you must drink at least <u>TWO</u> glasses of water. Then you can return to your clean diet. If you experience stomach discomfort during the four-hour waiting period, stick to salads for 24 hours. Some digestive systems can be quite cranky and sensitive. **The key to successfully breaking a fast is to do so slowly and always listen to your body.**

• If you chose **Half Week (IF)**: Break the fast with a 12-ounce glass of half fruit/half vegetable juice. Drink a glass of the juice every **FOUR** hours afterwards for an entire 24-hour cycle. No, if you are sleeping, you don't have to get up and drink. :-) If your tummy seems to be reacting well to the juice, then on the SECOND DAY you can have some sliced apples and pears for breakfast (*or any other fruit of your choice, barring citrus. They are too acidic and may cause discomf*ort). **FOUR** hours after you eat the fruit, if you feel well, have a basic salad with lettuce, tomatoes, cucumbers and/or carrots. For dressing, add a pinch of olive oil and sea salt. Chew the food well. **Chew, chew ... chew! Chew until the food dissolves in your mouth.**

TWO hours later, you can drink a glass of juice if you wish. For dinner, have a plate of **steamed veggies with a lean piece of fish or chicken, no larger than 8 ounces.** Chew the food well. Chew, chew ... chew!

Chew until the food dissolves in your mouth. If, at any time during this process, you start to feel stomach discomfort, <u>go back one phase for 12 hours</u>. In other words, if you had begun to eat fruit and your belly ached... return to only juice for 12 hours. If you ate steamed veggies with fish and your stomach protested, <u>return to salads for the next 12 hours</u>, and so on. If at the end of the second day your stomach has handled the re-feeding well, return to your clean diet ... you're done!

• If you chose **Seven Day (IF):** Purchase enough natural fruit and veggie juice to last you at least four days. Break the fast with an 8-ounce glass of half juice/half-water. Wait **FOUR** hours and have another watered-down glass of juice. If, in the afternoon, your belly is behaving, stop watering down the juice and have a full glass of the juice. Wait **FOUR** hours and drink another glass of the juice. Go to bed. If your stomach is doing well, continue to drink juice for at least another **FIVE HOURS** the second day. If you wake up at 7am, for example, keep drinking juice until <u>NOON</u>. You can then continue the re-feeding process from the ¥ symbol above.

• If you chose Combination (**IF**): Simply break each fast according to its corresponding instructions as specified above. That's it! <u>Note</u>: Regardless of which (**IF**) plan you have chosen, it is important that you drink at least one-gallon of water <u>EVERY DAY</u>. It is <u>NOT</u> enough to just drink the juice. You must continue to give the body sufficient liquids so that the digestive system can properly process the re-feeding.

Chapter 12
Your Breakthrough
Is At Hand

You now have absolutely <u>EVERYTHING</u> that you need to make your (**IF**) a success. <u>Take your time</u>; make sure you have enough food for your days off. Creating a new lifestyle is challenging but **possible and very rewarding**. I use the word *"creating"* because, indeed, that is what we are doing. Fasting can be rough, especially at first. If you have struggled, don't worry about it. The struggle is a normal and a fundamental part of <u>any</u> change and learning process.

The most important part is to <u>keep going</u>; <u>persist until you reach the breakthrough</u>. We are *"undoing"* years of negative habits. We are giving the mind and body an indivisible directive: **FORGE A NEW PATH!** This is not an overnight process, in most cases. The mind (*and body*) will resist change. If you are not steadfast and unrelenting, your goals and dreams can be squashed by **deceitful emotions including; self-hatred, condemnation, hopelessness, morbid guilt and shame.**

But, if you are <u>willing to walk past these feelings,</u> you will eventually – *and unequivocally* - attain your freedom

Here's an analogy that puts this truth in perspective: The mind and body are similar to a path created in the woods over many years. There are tall, wild weeds to the right and to the left. They are overgrown and full of sharp branches, puddles, poisonous plants and all types of slithering critters.

These *"untamed"* woods look <u>VERY</u> uninviting. But the path in the middle is <u>clear</u>, <u>safe</u> and <u>easy to trudge</u> because you have walked along it **your whole life**. <u>There are no weeds</u>. This path is secure, easy and very familiar. Anytime you want to cross the woods, do you walk through the overgrown, unfamiliar weeds or do you take the path that is already made? I would venture to say that you answered the latter. **So is the mind and body**. They will <u>ALWAYS</u> lead you towards that which is easy and familiar.

But **lasting change is never easy and familiar**. It is tough. It can be <u>scary</u> and <u>frustrating</u>. The process of change presented in this book is similar to starting a new path in the woods. To start this new path, you must enter the overgrown, unfamiliar and scary weeds. Entering this untamed part of the weeds will definitely not be as easy as simply walking through the path that is already made and you've used for years.

You may poke yourself with the weeds, you will probably have to cut through branches and other obstacles... you will become tired or maybe frustrated.

You may even have to confront a few serpents (*fear, doubt, unbelief*) and other dangerous animals (*procrastination, sloth, apathy*).

However, unless you want to continue to walk along the familiar path (*weight gain, poor health, dissatisfaction*), there really is <u>NO OTHER CHOICE</u> but to go through the temporary discomfort of creating a new one (*long-term weight loss, optimum health, self-esteem, reaching your goals and dreams*).

But you're not alone. There are many walking with you through the uncertain woods. Here I've given you the weapons and knowledge you need to go all the way and create that wonderful new path.

So there is much hope! Never back down! Your breakthrough is at hand...

God bless,

ROBERT DAVE JOHNSTON

Grab The Entire Collection:

Volume 1: The 'Permanent Weight Loss' Diet

Volume 2: The Intermittent Fasting Weight Loss Formula

Volume 3: How to Lose 30 Pounds (Or More) In 30 Days With Juice Fasting

Volume 4: Lose The Belly Fat Fast, And For Good!

Volume 5: Lose the Emotional Baggage: Transform Your Mind & Spirit With Fasting

Volume 6: How to Break a Fast (or Diet) and Keep The Weight Off

Volume 7: Compilation Volumes 1-6 -> Get All 5 For The Price Of 3!

Also by Robert Dave Johnston:

How To Lose Weight & Keep it Off By Transforming The Mind & Behaviors

Volume 1: How to Build a Rock-Solid Foundation That Supports Long-Term Weight Loss

Volume 2: How To Lose Weight & Keep it Off By Reprogramming The Subconscious Mind

Volume 3: How To Beat Diet Hunger and Junk Food Cravings

Volume 4: How to Escape the Diet "Time Trap" and Succeed in Weight Loss

Volume 5: How To Cheat On Your Diet (And Get Away With It)

Volume 6, Compilation: Get all 5 For The Price Of 3

Also By Robert Dave Johnston:

Detoxify Your Body, Lose Weight, Get Healthy & Transform Your Life

Volume 1- The 10-Day 'At Home' Colon Cleansing Formula

Volume 2- The 30-Day Kidney, Parasite & Liver Detox Weight Loss Method

Volume 3- Lose Weight Fast & Detoxify With Intermittent Fasting & At-Home Coffee Enemas

Volume 4 - Compilation: Get All 4 For The Price Of 2! Detoxify Your Body, Lose Weight, Get Healthy & Transform Your Life - Volumes 1-3

Don't forget to check the articles and growing health community at: FitnessThroughFasting.com

---